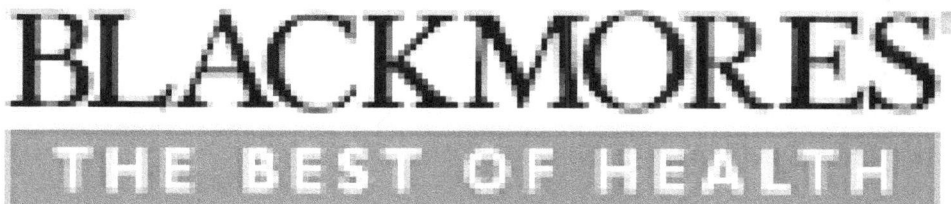

Blackmores showing the way:

The success of Blackmores supplement company

Blackmores showing the way:

The success of Blackmores supplement company

Contents

1. Introduction
2. Subjects/Themes
   - History of Blackmores
   - Growth and Production in Business/ Stockmarket/ Business-Management decisions
   - Asian-Chinese Market/Sponsorship
   - Importance of Information/Fight for Freedom
   - Blackmores compared to other supplement companies
   - Trend in Health and Fitness/Australian public use of supplements
   - Naturopathy versus General Medicine/Complimentary Medicines Industry/Health Organisations confronting each other
   - Company Culture /Employing People
   - Politics
   - Relationship and Friendships/Multicultural Links/Charity

- **University and Organisational influence**
- **Awards and Recognition**
- **Passion – Sailing and Helicopter/Childhood dream**

3. **Conclusion**
4. **Bibliography**

1. Introduction

The Blackmores company has been at the forefront of health supplements since the turn of the 19th Century. Blackmores helped bring supplements to the Australian and later global communities. The health food industry was largely unknown and understood in the early years. Maurice Blackmore set the foundation for himself and his son Marcus to learn, grow, improve, develop and further the Blackmore company and brand locally in Australia and overseas in regions like Asia-Pacific. The success of Blackmores has been nothing more than phenomenal. Lesser states that Blackmores is "the largest nutraceutical empire in the southern hemisphere." (Lesser, D. December 20, 2014) A customers has only got to walk into any chemist and or pharmacy to see the Blackmores products and or stand staring back at them in usually a highly visible section of the store. Blackmores would obviously have to pay large amounts of money for such strong in-store positioning. People have heard and or seen Blackmores products but not really know and understand the history and background of this influential, ground-breaking, successful and foundational health supplement companies.

2. Subjects/Themes

History of Blackmores

Maurice Blackmores was a somewhat rejected-illegitimate English immigrant to Australia in his 20s who had a powerful vision for health supplements. He was always well presented, wearing a jacket and tie. Maurice initially started with a focus on Naturopathy and Chiropractics, with some learning in America, and then branched into health food, opening a store in Brisbane in 1938. Maurice was also a "prolific writer and publisher." (Lesser, D. December 20, 2014) One of Maurice's books, 'Food Remedies', caused a throw-back by the Australian community because Maurice promoted the natural diet and its natural and medical value, and he questioned the competence of the medical profession. His family was against white sugar and white bread.

Health supplements were largely unknown by Australia and the rest of the world at this time, making way for the phenomenon of health supplements, including Blackmores vitamins, which were ahead of its time. This phenomenon occurred just at the start of World War II and the Vietnam War, being a gunnery officer and damaging his ears from such noise, making Maurice a somewhat scarred war veteran. It is actually amazing how Maurice survived the war to tell the tale and go to work on his visionary Blackmores company.

Growth and Production in Business/ Stockmarket/ Business-Management decisions

The alternative and complementary medicines industry "has grown 54 per cent in the past five years to be worth $3.5 billion in revenue a year and part of an estimated $138 billion annual global market." (Lesser, D. December 20, 2014) Blackmores is "driving growth in the general acceptance by the wider community of natural health and the trend towards wellbeing." (Heber, A. May 20, 2015). Blackmores had amassed about "8000 testimonials" throughout the years from his clinics. As a result, the Medical Acts Amendment Bill, brought in earlier by some doctors, politicians and press, was scrapped due to such evidence from Blackmores. Maurice and Marcus Blackmores now have a $2 billion company and "the most expensive stock on the Australian stockmarket." (Tasker, S-J. September 5, 2015) The Blackmores made the S&P/ASX 200 index after the company skyrocketed from $30 a share price to $100-to-$150 a share.

With this growth in supply-and-demand, Marcus Blackmores states how it can be difficult to just increase production to meet demands, for example, growing more herbs and making alternative-complementary medicine – "upping supply is not as easy as boosting production," states Marcus Blackmores (Heber, A. May 20, 2015). Blackmores made decisions to reduce costs, making a number of management decisions, including making David Fenlon managing director of Australia and NZ, as well as Christina Holgate as Chief Executive in November 2008.

Marcus states how the company did not predict this sort of growth, and had not seen growth like this – "We're struggling to make the product" (Heber, A. May 20, 2015). Heavy discounting of supplements in companies like Chemist Warehouse and Pharmacy for Less, with this reduction in pricing, meant profits of Blackmores were affected for a while. Fighting through this situation, Blackmores supplements were back in a big way. Blackmores Chief Executive since November 2008, Christina Holgate, "has tried to simplify the strategy and re-engage growth in the organisation." (Tasker, S-J. September 5, 2015)

Asian-Chinese Market/Sponsorship

One of the biggest, growing export markets for the Blackmores company is Asia. Blackmores "entered the Asian market 35 years ago." (Tasker, S-J. September 5, 2015) Strong growth in Blackmores has been "further enhanced by the rise of the middle class in China, who apparently are desperate to buy Australian vitamins." (Tasker, S-J. September 5, 2015). Asia's demand for western vitamins is between "$10bn to $15bn, with Australian companies accounting for about $200m of that." (Tasker, S-J. September 5, 2015). Actually, $200m is not much compared to a billion dollar Asian market; there is so much more Australia can do and accomplish. John Dwyer, for example, of the University of NSW and Friends OF Science Medicine (FSM), is critical of traditional Chinese medicine and reflexology.

Chinese medicine has been around for over 5000 years. Yet "just about every hospital in China has a reflexologist." (Lesser, D. December 20, 2014). Here is the Chinese supporting Australian-Blackmores supplements, and then there are people like John Dwyer criticising Chinese medicine; it sounds a bit unfair.

To further enhance Blackmores reach into Asia, the company is supporting the sport of Tennis. Female Chinese Tennis champion, Li Na, will be a sponsored ambassador for Blackmores to boost the company's profile in China. Blackmores will also be sponsoring the Australian Open in early 2016 where Li Na will be showcased. Blackmores has a "lucrative three-year deal with Asia's only Grand Slam winner, Lia Na, the retired ex-Australian Open women's champion." (Tabakoff, N. October 2, 2015)

Importance of Information/Fight for Freedom

Maurice and his son Marcus were ahead of their time in Australia, fighting for what was seen as far-fetched and radical during this period in the 1930s. The two individuals have pioneered, educated and serviced the Australian and overseas public by developing a whole system of healthcare with some of the first naturopathic colleges and professional associations and teachings. Maurice and Marcus fought hard early on to have health supplements and health phenomenon to be born and grow and progress.

Many of the world's leaders, intelligentsia, geniuses and learned people, like the Blackmores family, generally tended to have to fight for acceptance by specific and general worldwide publics.

Blackmores compared to other supplement companies

Although Blackmores has had this success, it is interesting and important, even powerful, to compare the product to other supplement companies in Australia and worldwide. Australian television program, Today Tonight, did a test of vitamins and nutritional supplements. According to Today Tonight, there is an enormous "30,000" supplement brands on the market, with "100 leading supplements available in Australia and New Zealand." (MyLifeChange, 13 June, 2008)

The questions then arises, which brand is better? Today Tonight disclosed a scientific study by Canadian and US biochemists. The scientists "evaluated and compared each brands formulations by separating and measuring each ingredient, with vitamins, minerals, antioxidants and other components...a range of issues were examined, with how absorbable the vitamins were, the range of vitamins and minerals that were in the tablet and whether they were in the appropriate amounts and form" (MyLifeChange, 13 June, 2008) It was called a 'wish list' of which brand had the ultimate multivitamin, or the best, by authors of 'Herbs and Natural Supplements', Dr. Lesley Braun, Pharmacist and Naturopath from the National Herbalists Association of Australia and Dr. Marc Cohen, Professor of Complementary Medicine at RMIT. (MyLifeChange, 13 June, 2008)

Some brands put some ingredients in, others put everything in, with the latter being a bit dangerous and limiting with its reaction with other things a person may ingest. Again, the validity of this study would certainly be in question, especially for these supplement companies like Blackmores having to protect, save and strengthen their brand image, reputation and results.

Some of the better supplements are really found at supermarkets and pharmacies. These supplements are actually found online, directly from naturopaths and herbalists and networking-multilevel marketing companies. Networking company, USANA, topped the list with its "Health Sciences Essentials scoring a very high 74 per cent." (MyLifeChange, 13 June, 2008) In fact, this USANA product scored well above the rest of supplements, with the closest, "Solgar Opnium" scoring 56.5 per cent. Amway, another prominent Networking company, had its "Nutriway Double X" at "27.3", in 9th position. It seemed Blackmores Women's multivitamins were the best for Blackmores, scoring "14.1 percent, 13.4 per cent and13.3 per cent". The Blackmores Men's multi-vitamin scored "6.2 per cent" and Blackmores Multivitamin with Ginko for 55+ "3 per cent". (MyLifeChange, 13 June, 2008)

Firstly, this list is just multivitamins, and not the whole range of each of the brands. Secondly, these are huge results and differences when each of the brands are compared to the extent that the accuracy of the results would be in question. Blackmores would be somewhat dissatisfied with the results, but also other more expensive and supposedly stronger-performing brands would be quite upset at these findings.

Trend in Health and Fitness/Australian public use of supplements

Blackmores can be wholeheartedly recognised as one of the primary instigators behind the current health and fitness phenomenon in Australia and around the world. People in general know and understand more about health and fitness than ever before, including previous generations (War-time populations, Baby Boomers and Generation X). According to Lesser, "an estimated 70 per cent of Australians are regular users of a natural healthcare product." (Lesser, D. December 20, 2015) This 70 per cent is an astounding amount, considering there are people like John Dwyer about who promote to the general public that they are against the alternative and complementary industry. The general public are growingly becoming aware that a healthy diet alone is not substantial without some form of health food supplementation.

Mother Nature has blessed the human race of containing many nutrients that are exactly or closely replicated in supplements like Blackmores and others. It is true some people especially from older generations, have lived to old-elderly age with just food alone and no supplements and some form of movement-exercise. However the risk is there, with current and older generations, dying younger or older, with media news reporting ad hoc sickness, illness and death Son of Maurrice, Marcus, for example ingests a multivitamin and omega-3 fish oil every day. According to Lesser, "surveys have shown many Australians are spending $80 or more a month on supplements." (Lesser, D. December 30, 2014).

This health and fitness trend is unearthing dissatisfied and disillusioned practitioners and members of the public who are sick and tired of ill-proper health food and services. The health system, previously and currently is still largely segregated and categorised that tends to not work in together to strengthen and maximise health products and services like Blackmores. Examples are Australians Cardiologist-Health presenter and Researcher, Dr. Ross Walker, American General Practitioner-Health Presenter and Researcher, Dr. Russell Blaylock, Australian General Practitioner-Researcher Dr. Sandra Cabot and former Australian Christian nun-turned Naturopathic-Reiki practitioner, Ethel. Dr. Ross Walker has published a strongly influential material, with book 'Live Fast, Die Young' and a talk-presentation, 'Balance is Everything'.

Similar phenomenon's occurring at this same time, with technology and information and the Internet, helped fuel and quickly spread the health and fitness trend for Blackmores. People can quickly educate and inform and purchase endless health food and services with general web-sites like Ebay and Amazon and the plethora of health food and service web-sites. These web-sites cut out the middle-men like chemists and pharmacies like Chemist Warehouse and Pharmacy for Less.

Naturopathy versus General Medicine/Complimentary Medicines Industry/Health Organisations confronting each other

The battle between Naturopathy and General Medicine existed in Maurice Blackmores time, and surprisingly, still continues in today's global society. Maurice Blackmores views were considered radical in the 1930s, with interpretations on "natural health, preventative medicine, the environment and recycling...in treating illness and maximising health." (Blackmores.com.au) People either concentrated solely on standard food, some exercise and movement, and visiting their General Practitioner-

Doctor and being given medicine, without seeing the need for health food supplements. A number of GPs are not generally educated about health food supplements and the need for them.

The line is that, 'You get all your nutritional needs from your diet.' This may have been the case in previous years, but the scourge of modern society involves poor farming practices and preservatives in food, working long hours, both partners in a relationship working, pollution, technology and social media, more reliance on medication, and so on. Maurice Blackmore, regarded by many as the father of Australian naturopathy, was even quoted as stating, 'So why do patients only come to seek my advice after they've been t five doctors without any results?'

There are health organisations representing Naturopathy and health food supplements and Blackmores and General Medicine and General Practitioners that are against each other. While Blackmore established the Complimentary Medicine Association (formerly National Nutritional Association of Australia), John Dwyer, professor of medicine at the University of NSW made the Friends of Science in Medicine (FSM) opposing Blackmore and his stance. Dwyer attacked the complementary and alternative medicines industry, endeavouring to have certain courses removed from higher education. Dwyer emailed the National Health and Medical Research Council (NHMRC) wanting to see what he calls 'nonsense' courses removed, such as "homeopathy, reflexology, kinesiology, healing touch therapy, chiropractic, acupuncture, iridology, crystal therapy, reiki, energy medicine and traditional Chinese medicine be removed from tertiary courses." (Lesser, D. December 20, 2014)

Dwyer went on to state that, "from a scientific, clinical point of view, alternative medicine has got very little use for people to stay healthy or to help them with their health problems." (Lesser, D. December 20, 2014). The NHMRC ended up agreeing with Dwyer, after a review into the complementary and alternative medicine industry and "concluded there was no reliable evidence for its effectiveness in treating health conditions" (Lesser, D. December 20, 2014). John Dwyer has made an art from being a critic of the industry. However, Blackmores and his supporters casted great doubt on the review process of the NHMRC review process. The doctors mentioned previously, Dr. Ross Walker, Dr. Russell Blaylock, Dr. Sandra Cabot, Ethel and Dr. Duke Johnson from the Nutriway Institute have all provided strong evidence supporting the use of alternative and complementary medicines. So something is wrong here.

Company Culture /Employing People

Blackmores is a public company that "employs over 530 [up to 900] people across Australia, New Zealand and Asia." (University of Western Sydney, News Centre) Marcus' father, Maurice, instilled strong core values in him from young about hard-work, overcoming adversity and supporting the alternative and complementary industry, and this has flowed down to the staff and employees – "that's a depth of belief, it's purpose and passion." (Tasker, S-J. September 5, 20-15). Maurice and Marcus Blackmores place high value on their staff and employees.

With the success of the Blackmores company, being bigger and more successful, Marcus Blackmore states how, "you can afford to employ bigger and better people." (Heber, A. May 20, 2015). According to Tasker, "a recent employee survey found that 94% of the 900 staff 'had a strong commitment to the company' " (Tasker, S-J. September 5, 2015). To highlight this acknowledgement of Blackmores' staff, they received a "bonus of six weeks pay...staff now get 7.5% plus an extra 2.5% if the company achieves its budget."(Tasker, S-J. September 5, 2015)

Politics

Marcus Blackmore, the son of Maurice, faced industry and political adversity from people like University of NSW John Dwyer of Friends of Science in Medicine (FSM). Dwyer and the like questioned and criticized the worth and affects of Blackmores and the alternative and complementary medicines industry. Australian politicians, along with doctors and the press, joined Dwyer in a way by previously bringing in the Medical Acts Amendments Bill. However, Blackmores 8000 testimonials from his patients experiences, and sheer hard work, at his clinics provided some fight back against Dwyer, politicians and the like. Lesser highlights how Marcus stated, "if it wasn't for those strong political connections there wouldn't be any naturopaths in Australia." (Lesser, D. December 20, 2014).

The most powerful thing Marcus Blackmore did was three years ago, in 2011, where he made a presentation to federal politicians and bureaucrats to argue the case for natural medicine. There were senior Labor and Liberal party politicians there at this presentation, including "Simon Crean, Julie Bishop, Phillip Ruddock and Peter Dutton."(Lesser, D. December 20, 2014). The presentation flowed on after a report by Access Economics came out "showing that millions of dollars in healthcare costs could be saved if complementary medicine was more widely used." (Lesser, D. December 20, 2014) Would one believe that "all the bottles [Blackmores showcased that day] went, according to Blackmores Chief Executive Christine Holgate."

Blackmores was only in the building a short time when politicians from all walks congratulated him and shook his hands. Australian Federal Prime Minister at the time, Tony Abbott, was believed to be taking Blackmores supplements, as was Jillian Skinner, NSW Minister for Health. Skinner stated that "nothing much could be done about her macular degeneration than the diet and taking supplements." (Lesser, D. December 20, 2014)

Relationship and Friendships/Multicultural Links/Charity

Maurice and Marcus Blackmores have amassed many allies, supporters and friends along the way since their early days in Australia. The Blackmores have "always supported their close friends." According to Lesser, Marcus Blackmores has "more friends than most people could collect in three lifetimes." Lesser goes on to highlight how "his [Marcus Blackmores] network of friends is a testament to something far more enduring than mere business prowess." (Lesser, D. December 20, 2014) Marcus donates money to needy people and worthy causes and invests a large amount of time into people and causes.

For example, Marcus helped people in Samoa, with schools damaged in the 2009 tsunami, and is an honorary chief. Lesser states how Petrea King made the comment about Marcus, that "there's no one quite like Blackmore in Australia." (Lesser, D. December 20, 2014). Marcus Blackmores shows that not all rich people are greedy and selfish in the world.

Marcus, who was 68 years of age at the time, in 2013 recently invited 150 friends to Hamilton Island for a three-day celebration of his wedding to Caroline

Furlong, his partner of 15 years (Lesser, D. December 20, 2014). Marcus stated about his wedding that sometimes decisions, like his wedding, can take some time. Marcus also has a son, Alexander (Aly) Borromeo, from his former marriage to his Filipino-Phillipines mother. Aly was brought up in the Philippines and was present at Marcus recent 2013 wedding. Aly is the former captain of the Philippines national football (Soccer) team.

University and Organisational influence

Marcus Blackmores "holds an Honorary Doctorate from Southern Cross University for distinguished leadership in complementary medicines in Australia." (University of Western Sydney, News Centre). Marcus admitted he had failed at university earlier in his life, starting a Science degree at Queensland University only to fail in the first year. Other popular and successful school drop outs in business, like Marcus Blackmores are Australian Dick Smith, Britain Richard Branson of Virgin and American Bill Gates of Microsoft. Marcus is also Chairman of the Heart Research Institute and Director of the National Maritime Museum.

Marcus went on to make the point that "life is a continuum of personal challenges of both achievement and by failure." (University of Western Sydney, News Centre). An example of this was the initial rejection, questioning and criticism of Blackmores and the alternative and complementary industry, only to have it accepted later on. Marcus stated how "it is not so much what you have learned but how you have learned that will be important in later life"… "Education is what survives when what has been learned has been forgotten"… "Much of what you have learned will be irrelevant in 10 years' time"…"Knowledge is more freely available to individuals than ever before"… "Google gets billions of searches per day. Knowledge is infinite in its nature."

Marcus also reflected on previous war times like Anzac Day where many individuals fought for Australia's and the world's democracy and freedoms. Businesses like Blackmores create wealth, better living standards, goodwill and understanding, values, responsible behaviour, mutual respect, tolerance, understanding, corporate social investment and 'living one's dreams' (University of Western Sydney, News Centre).

Awards and Recognition

First and foremost, Blackmores is "the largest nutraceutical empire in the southern hemisphere," as stated in the Introduction (Lesser, D. December 20, 2014) The Blackmores.com.au site states that over 80 years of Blackmores has brought a number of awards and recognition. During 2014 and 2013, there is the "Readers Digest survey winner...New Headquarters for Blackmores Asia and China and Macau launch...Blackmores partnering with health and fitness expert Michelle Bridges...Australian environmental packaging covenant recognition and reducing carbon emissions..Education accreditation from Royal Australian College of General Practitioners and Australian Pharmacy Council...Blackmores honoured by Heart Research Institute...Blackmores partnership with Quest for Life organisation to help local communities." (Blackmores.com.au)

Passion – Sailing and Helicopter/Childhood dream

These days, it is important for people of all walks of life to have some form of hobby and interest outside of their mainstream activities. Marcus has these such hobbies and interests in sailing and boats and plane and helicopters. Marcus' passion provides a great outlet from his busy activities and schedule with the Blackmores company. According to Lesser, Marcus Blackmores has six vessels (boats), including a Palm Beach 50 boat moored at his private jetty at Sydney's Pittwater. With Marcus' love of water, he had the childhood dream of being a ferryman. Marcus for example assisted Kay Cottee in 1988, aboard her Blackmores First Lady boat, to make Cottee's historic 189-day solo voyage around the world.

Marcus also enjoys planes and helicopters, where at 60 years of age he learned to pilot his "French-made Squirrel jet-engine helicopter which he stations at Sydney's Mascot airport." (Lesser, D. December 20, 2014) Marcus once flew himself and a friend by helicopter to Dubbo to watch a music festival about Johnny Cash. With Marcus' involvement in the war, and love of boats and planes, he is vice-chairman of the Defence Support Reserves Council. (Lesser, D. December 20, 2014)

3. Conclusion

With all that has happened to the Blackmores company, both good and bad, it will be interesting to see how the business fairs, now and in the future. Blackmores was first around when the health and fitness trend and the alternative and complimentary medicines industry was initially moving. Now, today, Blackmores can hold its head high for being a true performer, leader and influencer in such an industry, and related areas, such as staff and employees, friendships, charity and sponsorship. There looks like to be so much more left for Blackmores to do and achieve in the coming years.

4. Bibliography

- Blackmores.com.au, 'Heritage and History', 'Leadership: A series of firsts', 'Over 80 years of Blackmores'

- Heber, Alex. (May 20, 2015) 'Look how much Blackmores shares have soared since its CEO told the board he was buying a yacht', <u>Business Insider</u>

- Lesser, David. (December 20, 2014) 'Marcus Blackmore: the medicine man', <u>Sydney Morning Herald</u>

- Tabakoff, Nick (October 2, 2015) 'Vitamin king Marcus Blackmore rides a $25 billion rocket', <u>The Daily Telegraph</u>

- Tasker, Sarah-Jane (September 5, 2015) 'Blackmores a $2bn success as shares pass $100', <u>The Australian</u>

- University of Western Sydney, 'News Centre: Marcus C Blackmore AM, Chairman, Blackmores Ltd'

- Wellings, Helen (13 June, 2008) 'Today Tonight Test of Vitamins and Nutritional Supplements, <u>MyLifeChange</u>